Deliciously
Ella
Smoothies
& Juices

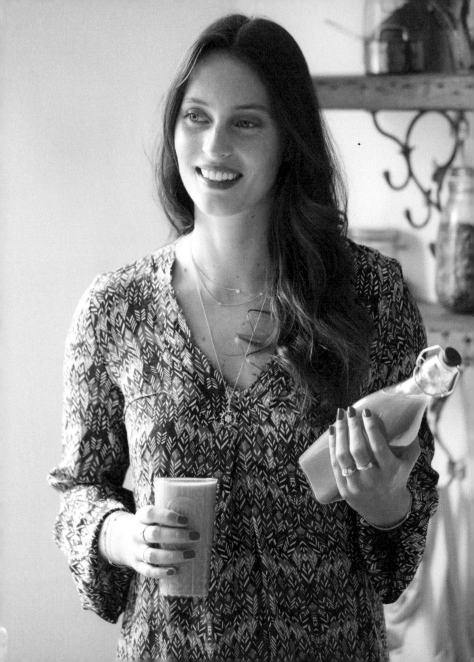

Deliciously Ella

Smoothies & Juices

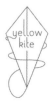

yellow kite

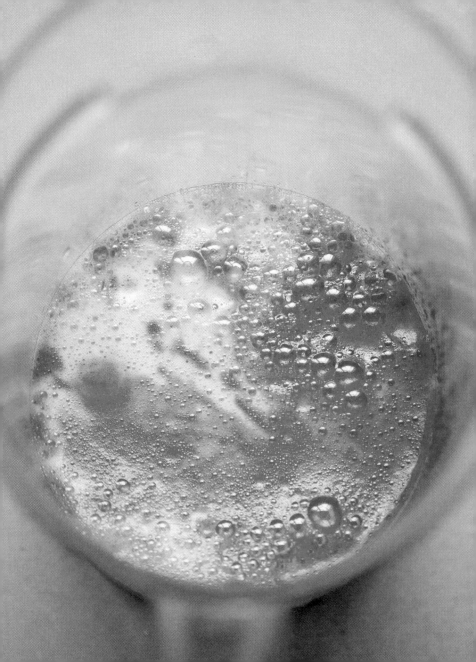

CONTENTS

INTRO

Both smoothies and juices are a big part of my weekly routine. I love how easy they make it to load up on fruit and veg, especially when I'm really busy. Every week my diary seems to get more and more packed and I don't always have the time to make the meals that I'd like, so I'm constantly looking for simple ways to make sure I still get a variety of nutrients in my diet and blending and juicing is a quick way to do this. I also find that the better I feel, the more productive I am, so during crazy periods I try to make one of these every morning to take with me on the go. That way I know I've had three or four portions of fruit and veg before my day has even started, so I don't have to worry about getting so much in at every other meal, and I start the day on a positive note that inspires me to take care of myself, even when I'm totally non-stop!

SMOOTHIES VS JUICES
I'll go into more detail about the differences between the two in the chapter introductions that follow, but the main thing to note now is that smoothies are thicker, creamier and contain the fibre from the ingredients, whereas juices are smooth, thin liquids that have had the majority of their pulp removed. This means that smoothies are more filling, especially as you can also load them up with other ingredients, like oats and almond butter.

As a result, I tend to have smoothies as a whole meal – normally at breakfast. I find I can make them just as satisfying as anything else I'd eat for that meal, but they're often a lot quicker and easier to take with me. However, I tend to enjoy my juice alongside something else. If I have a juice with breakfast, for example, I'll make a bowl of creamy porridge with banana and nut butter to have with it, or a chia pudding with coconut yogurt and granola. Alternatively I fill a big tumbler with juice and keep it on my desk to enjoy throughout the day, as it's lovely to have something refreshing to sip on between meals.

There's a tendency to want to go totally green with these drinks, as we're always hearing so much about the benefits of green juice, but don't feel that you need to love drinking hardcore veggie mixes immediately: it's normal not to enjoy sipping on broccoli and coriander straight away! I certainly didn't like those no-fruit mixes to start with and needed sweetness to enjoy the tastes (I really thought a 'mean green' combo tasted a bit like grass the first time around!), so don't worry if you're the same. I was used to eating pretty processed, overly-sweetened cereal for breakfast and I wasn't able to go from that to blended kale and cucumber, I needed frozen chunks of mango, pineapple and lots of nut butter to get used to the concept. I always added apple to my veggie juices until my taste buds started to change – but that took a while.

It's OK to start your smoothies and juices journey off gently. I think for most people it's definitely a case of building up and letting your taste buds adapt. If you're already making green mixes, but not really enjoying them because they're a bit hardcore, then ease off and let yourself enjoy some sweeter blends rather than forcing liquid kale down you! Yes, green juice is great, but it's much better to make something that you love – that satisfies you and that you want to incorporate into your life – than it is to make something that you secretly hate and takes you hours to drink while you wish you were eating biscuits instead! Remember, there's

no rush on your health journey, we all have to start somewhere and a healthy lifestyle should be enjoyable, fun and sustainable – it's not something where you should have to hold your nose to be able to swallow!

So please bear that in mind as you go through the book, and feel free to adapt recipes to make them work for you. Add extra apple to a juice, or a couple of dates to a smoothie, just make sure you enjoy every sip. That's how I was able to make them a part of my routine.

There's a great mix of recipes in this book, covering all my favourite smoothies and juices from the last few years, ranging from my new love of green-everything to my comforting blends filled with frozen banana, nut butter and cacao, as well as some lovely refreshing combinations. I hope you all enjoy making them as much as I do, and once you see how easy they are, I'm sure they'll become a natural part of your life, too.

Ella x

WEIGHTS OF FRUIT & VEG

Fruit and vegetables vary a lot in size, so I thought it would be helpful to include here the list of weights that I used for each recipe, to give you a rough idea of the measurements needed to get the right flavour and quantity.

Top tips: try to use really ripe fruit; the riper a banana or mango etc. is, the better a smoothie will taste.

Sweetness levels can vary a lot though, so feel free to adapt the recipes depending on the quality and freshness of the ingredients you're using on any given day.

It's a great idea to store very ripe bananas, peeled and cut into slices, in a sealed bag in your freezer. That way they're ready to go and you'll get the best flavour in your smoothie.

Apple 1 medium = 150g
Avocado 1 medium = 160g
Banana 1 medium = 100g
Beetroot 1 small = 110g
Blueberries 1 handful = 70g
Broccoli 1 medium head = 400g
Carrot 1 medium = 80–90g
Cashew nuts 1 handful = 35g
Celery 1 stick = 45g
Cucumber 1 medium = 340g
Fennel 1 medium bulb = 280g
Ginger (root) 1 thumb-sized chunk = 25–35g
Grapefruit 1 medium = 350g
Grapes 1 small bunch = 135g
Greens (kale, spinach and so on) 1 handful = 30g
Herbs 1 small handful = 10–15g
Lemon 1 medium = 60g
Lemon grass 1 stalk = 12g
Lime 1 medium = 40g

Mango 1 medium, peeled and pitted = 340g
Melon 1 honeydew = 950g–1kg
Orange 1 medium = 150g
juice of 1 medium = 100ml
Papaya 1 medium, peeled and deseeded = 300g
Passion fruit 1 medium, flesh only (out of skin) = 25–30g
Peach 1 medium, pitted = 140g
Pear 1 medium = 180g
Pineapple 1 medium = 850–900g
Raspberries 1 handful = 70g
Strawberries 6 berries, hulled = 90g
Sweet potato 1 medium = 270g
Tomato 1 medium = 120g
Turmeric 1 thumb-sized chunk = 22g

… and a note on liquid measures
For my juice and smoothie recipes, 1 glass = 400ml

NUT MILKS & BUTTERS 101

As there are lots of nut milks and butters in this book, I just wanted to share a little recap on how to make them, so you can make them at home if you'd like. They normally have more flavour than store-bought options, so it's definitely worth trying if you have the time. The ratio of ingredients given for the nut milk below makes a lovely creamy milk. You can alter the thickness though, by adding more or less water, to get the perfect texture for you.

TO MAKE 1 LITRE OF NUT MILK

Soak 200g of nuts (normally almonds, cashews or hazelnuts) in water overnight, or for about six hours.

Drain the soaking water, then blend with 1 litre of fresh water.

Pour the mix through a nut milk bag or a jelly bag (both available online), squeezing it to get all the liquid out.

Store in an airtight container in the fridge for about five days. Always use plant-based milks chilled in your smoothies; for some reason the drinks taste far nicer when everything is good and cold!

TIP If you have a nut allergy, replace all nut butters with tahini or pumpkin seed butter, and all nut milks with oat or brown rice milk.

TO MAKE 1 JAR (ABOUT 170G) OF NUT BUTTER

Roast 250g of nuts (I normally use almonds or cashews) for about ten minutes in an oven preheated to 200°C (fan 180°C); keep an eye on them and do not let them burn! Leave to cool.

Place in a food processor and blend for ten minutes or so, until a creamy mix forms. It always takes longer than you think to create a great texture, so be patient with it. This does need a food processor, rather than a blender, as it may break your blender!

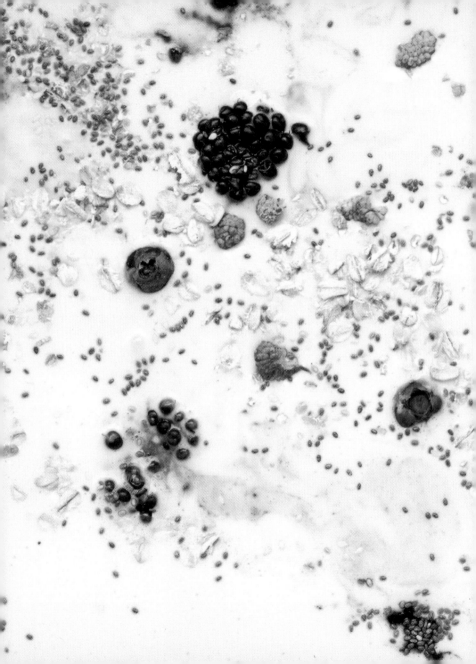

SMOOTHIES

SMOOTHIES INTRO

This chapter will take you through all my favourite smoothies. I want to share a little information with you here about making smoothies and – of course – my best tips and tricks, too.

Smoothies are made using a blender, which mixes the ingredients into a liquid. As a result, smoothies are thicker and more filling than juices, as they contain all the pulp from the fruit and veg, plus any extra ingredients that you add. Nothing is removed when you make a smoothie, it's simply all broken down.

The great thing about blending is that you can use pretty much any fruit or veg, plus a whole host of other ingredients. I add everything from oats to dates, sesame seeds, nut butter, chia seeds, tahini, cacao powder, coconut yogurt, coconut oil, hemp seeds, spices and herbs to my blender, plus anything else I can find in my cupboard! There's no limit to what you can throw in, so you can get really creative. This flexibility means you have a great variety of flavour options, so your smoothie can be totally different from one day to the next.

I freeze a lot of the fruit and veg I'm going to use in my smoothies, from chunks of banana and mango to spinach, kale and berries. Not only does freezing mean you've always got your ingredients ready to go, frozen fruit also gives smoothies a lovely creamy texture and is the best way to make your smoothie cold without having to water it down with ice.

All you need to make a smoothie is some kind of liquid base – I normally use nut milk, oat milk or coconut water – and then you can throw in any other ingredients. It's really so simple. The more liquid you add, the runnier it will be, so if you use just a splash you'll end up with a thick, creamy smoothie bowl that you can top with crunchy bites of granola, extra dollops of nut butter, fresh berries and anything else.

My favourite thing about smoothies is how quick they are to make. They also require minimal washing up, which is a massive bonus, especially if you're rushed in the mornings and need something easy to take with you. Just chuck your ingredients in, blend, pour into a to-go cup and quickly rinse your blender. At a push you can be ready to go, smoothie in hand, in just two minutes. So these are ideal for busy mums and dads and those of us who need to disappear out the door when it's still dark!

A FEW TIPS ON BUILDING A SMOOTHIE

1 Add some chilled liquid: plant-based milk, coconut water, cucumber or carrot juice and so on.

2 Add a fibrous piece of fruit or veg: I find avocados, bananas and mangos work best, but pears and peaches are also good. Without one of these, the result will be watery rather than creamy.

Steps 1 and 2 above are pretty essential; those below are optional (I normally only do a few of them).

3 Add extra fruit: strawberries, raspberries, blueberries, blackberries, apples, lime, lemon...

4 Add some greens. It's easy to sneak greens into a smoothie, even a sweet one, as the other flavours will mask the taste. Baby leaf spinach blends really easily and has the mildest flavour.

5 Add extras to make the smoothie creamier and more filling: nut butters, oats, hemp seeds, tahini, chia seeds and coconut yogurt are great for this.

6 Add extra flavour: spices like cinnamon, vanilla, ginger, cardamom and turmeric; fresh herbs like mint and basil; or try cacao powder, matcha or a pinch of salt.

7 Add sweetness if you want something more indulgent: honey and dates are my go-tos.

8 Add ice if you want it, then put the lid on the blender and blend until smooth.

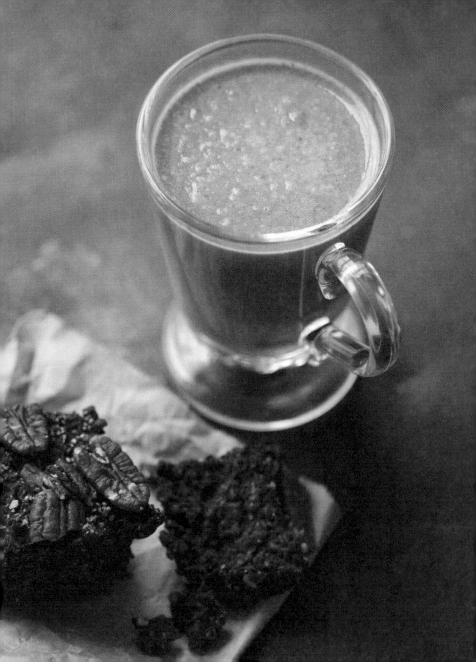

CHOCOLATE HAZELNUT MYLK

A wonderfully indulgent, chocolatey smoothie that sates my afternoon sweet tooth every time. If I feel that four o'clock energy slump coming on, I often make this to perk me up again and always really enjoy it. The mix of sweet hazelnut milk, cacao and orange zest is just a dream!

SERVES 1

½ glass of chilled hazelnut milk (200ml)
1 teaspoon date syrup
1 ripe banana, peeled and frozen (100g)
½ teaspoon sesame seeds
1 teaspoon cacao powder
1 teaspoon almond butter
1 teaspoon finely grated unwaxed
   orange zest
tiny pinch of salt (just a very small pinch,
   it won't taste good otherwise!)

Place all the ingredients in a blender. Blend until smooth and creamy.

TIP Make frozen nut butter cubes in silicone ice trays, it's a great way to portion it out and a really nice way to make a smoothie colder, creamier and more refreshing.

ALMOND, HEMP &
BLUEBERRY BOWL

One of my favourite breakfasts after a
workout. I'll make the bowl and then load
it up with toppings to add extra flavour and
texture. The mix of almond butter, hemp,
banana and avocado makes it so thick and
creamy, while the blueberries make it the
most beautiful colour and the cinnamon
adds a lovely flavour.

SERVES 1

¼ avocado (40g)
2 tablespoons almond butter
1 ripe banana, peeled and frozen (100g)
small handful of frozen blueberries
  (about 20g)
1 tablespoon hulled hemp seeds
½ teaspoon ground cinnamon
2–3 tablespoons chilled almond milk

Pit and peel the avocado, put everything
into a blender, then blend until smooth
and creamy. You may need to stop the
blender once or twice and mix it all
around, as there isn't much liquid here,
so ingredients can sometimes get stuck.

TIP Frozen berries of all kinds are easy to
come by and great to have on hand for
mixing into smoothies; they're normally
cheaper too.

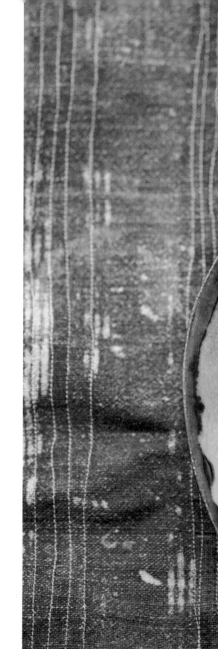

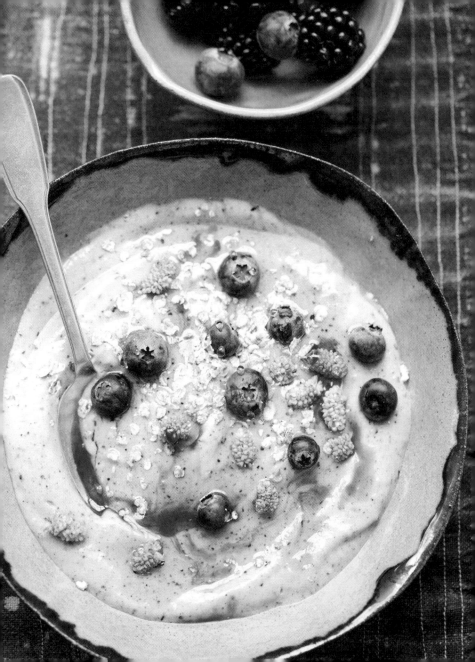

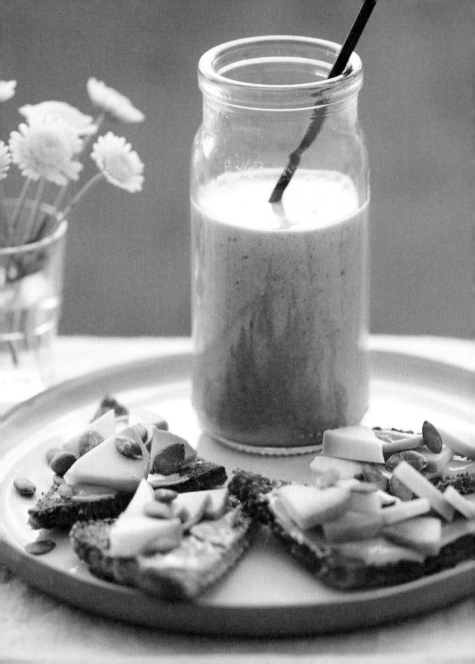

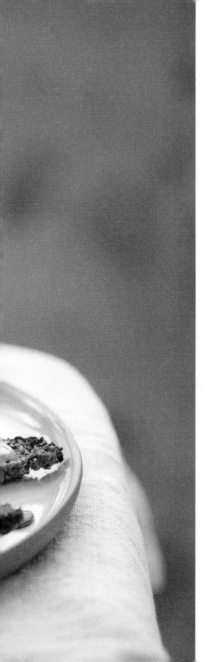

CASHEW & COFFEE

This cashew and coffee blend is so delicious. I'm not a huge coffee drinker, but when it tastes this good I really love it. It's a great breakfast option if you need a bit of help waking up, and you can even skip the banana and use the rest of the mix like a milk on your granola alongside the drink. It makes a fantastic afternoon pick-me-up, too.

SERVES 1

½ glass of chilled cashew milk (200ml)
½–1 ripe banana, peeled and frozen
  (50–100g; I use ½ for a snack,
  1 for breakfast)
1 teaspoon cashew butter
1 teaspoon tahini
1 shot of espresso coffee
½ teaspoon ground cinnamon
tiny pinch of salt
1 medjool date, pitted and chopped
  (optional)

Simply add everything to a blender.

Blend until smooth and creamy.

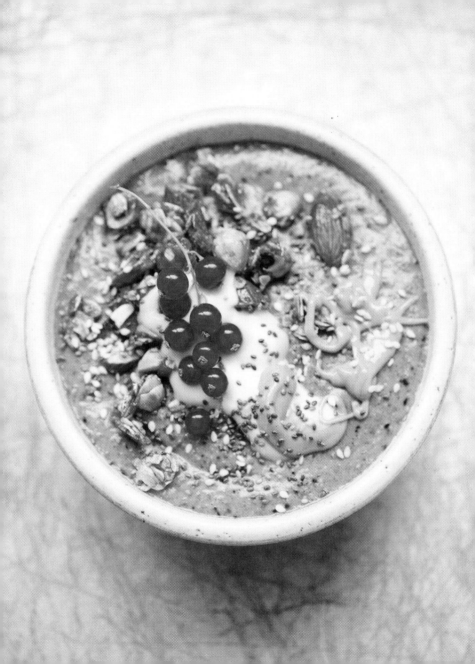

CREAMY MANGO & STRAWBERRY BOWL

My husband's favourite recipe in this book. We have it together on weekends a lot and really enjoy it every time. The thing I love about this recipe is that it makes an amazingly fruity, creamy mix that I can pile high with mountains of home-made oaty granola, which tastes incredible mixed in. It's a bit like using a fruit yogurt with cereal, but more flavoursome and with lots more fresh produce that should help you to feel great.

If you want this to be a thinner smoothie, rather than a bowl, then leave out the oats and add a splash of your favourite plant-based milk.

SERVES 1

½ ripe mango, peeled and pitted, preferably frozen (170g)
2 heaped teaspoons coconut yogurt
6 strawberries, hulled (90g)
handful of blueberries (about 70g)
1 tablespoon chia seeds
1 teaspoon vanilla powder
1 medjool date, pitted and chopped
2 tablespoons oats

Place all the ingredients in a blender and blend until smooth and creamy. You may need to stop the blender and mix the ingredients around once or twice if your blender isn't really powerful, as there isn't much liquid here, so ingredients can get stuck.

Top with anything you like. I love a swirl of nut butter, granola, coconut yogurt and berries.

TIP Hull strawberries, then cut into thirds or quarters before freezing in a sealed bag. This makes blending them so much easier; whole frozen strawberries are like little bricks! Frozen mango is easy to find in supermarkets too.

TROPICAL PAPAYA, MANGO & LIME

This smoothie instantly transports me to warm climates and sunny beaches, which makes me so happy every time I make it... especially on a grey Monday morning in London! The mix of papaya, frozen mango, lime, cinnamon and coconut water can brighten up any day and always tastes amazing. The trick with this blend is to make sure the fruit is really ripe, as that makes a huge difference to the flavour, so it's worth letting the fruit sit in your kitchen until it's perfectly sweet rather than using it up straight away.

NUT FREE

SERVES 1

½ ripe papaya, peeled and deseeded (150g)
handful of frozen mango chunks (85g)
juice of 1 lime
½ teaspoon ground cinnamon
¾ glass of chilled coconut water, preferably raw and unpasteurised (300ml)
1 teaspoon honey (optional, you should only need this if you like it extra sweet)

Place all the ingredients in a blender and blend until smooth and creamy.

TIP Freeze any leftover produce you may have to make smoothies, it's a great way to prevent waste. I freeze all fruit and veg I'm going to use for smoothies, from spinach to mango, pineapple and berries. Plus buying frozen ingredients in the first place can often work out cheaper than fresh, so is a great way to save money.

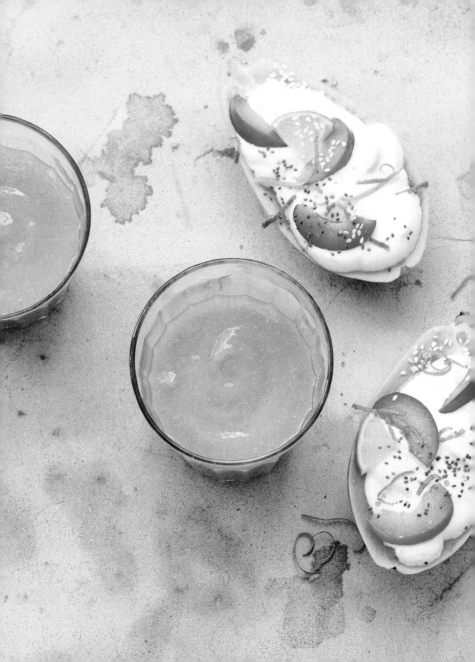

FROZEN RASPBERRY, PEACH & ORANGE

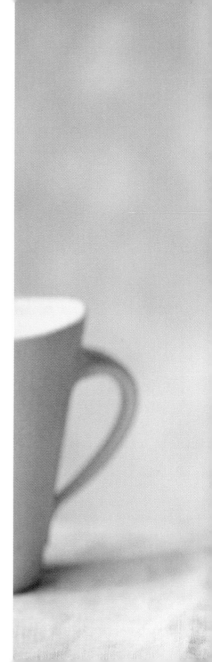

This smoothie reminds me of English summers. I tend only to make it when peaches are in season, as they're much easier to find then and – most importantly – taste so much better, so I look forward to making it every winter! This is a lovely drink to make and share with friends on a warm day, or to enjoy as an afternoon snack to sate your sweet tooth and keep you going until dinner.

NUT FREE

SERVES 1

2 oranges (300g)
1 ripe peach (140g)
handful of frozen raspberries (70g)
½ ripe banana, peeled and frozen (50g),
   or a second peach, if you prefer
1 tablespoon oats

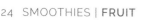

Squeeze the juice out of the oranges using a citrus press (you should get about 200ml), and pour it into a blender. Cut the peach into the blender around the stone, discarding the stone (you can keep the skin on, as it's so thin it blends well). Add the remaining ingredients and blend until smooth and creamy.

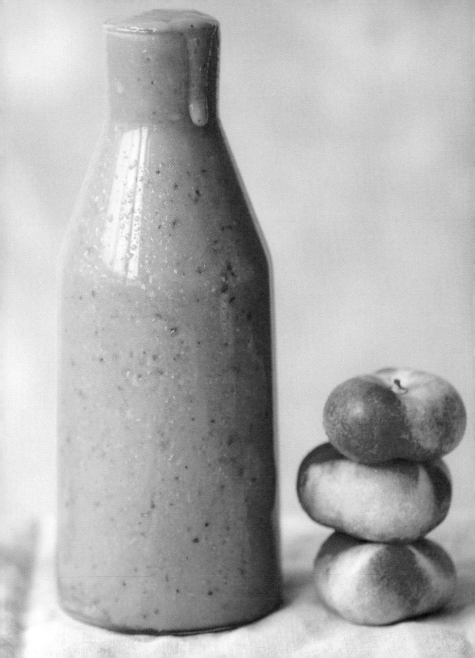

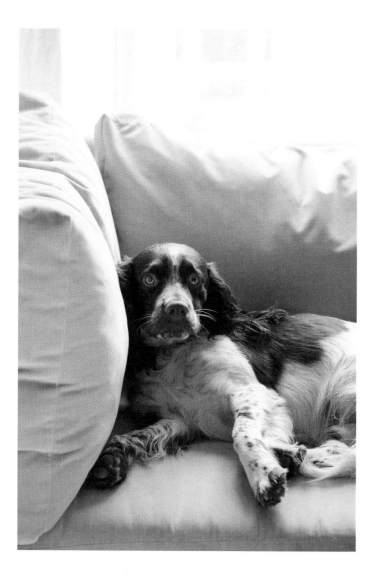

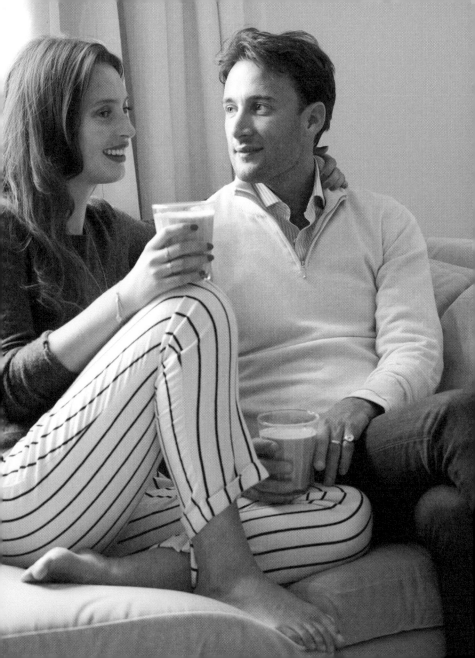

GREEN DREAM

One of my go-to breakfast smoothies, I absolutely love starting my day with a big glass of this. Pineapple is one of my favourite foods, so anything including it is a winner for me; I love how it's used here to create a subtle sweetness, while the avocado and almond milk make this creamy, the spinach ups the greens and the coconut oil, lemon and ginger add lots of flavour.

SERVES 1

½ avocado (80g)
handful of fresh or frozen spinach (30g)
a few chunks of pineapple (80g)
1 teaspoon coconut oil
squeeze of lemon juice
slice of fresh ginger, peeled (5g)
½ glass of chilled almond milk, or any
    other plant-based milk (200ml)

Peel and pit the avocado, place in a blender then add all the other ingredients and blend until smooth.

TIP Add protein powder, hemp seeds, tahini or almond butter to any smoothie after a workout, to help you refuel.

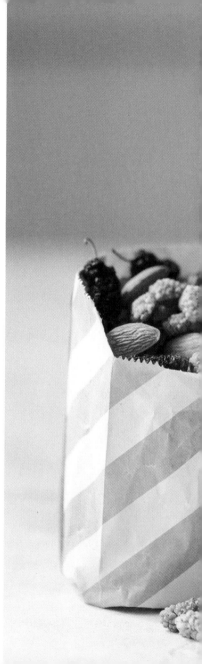

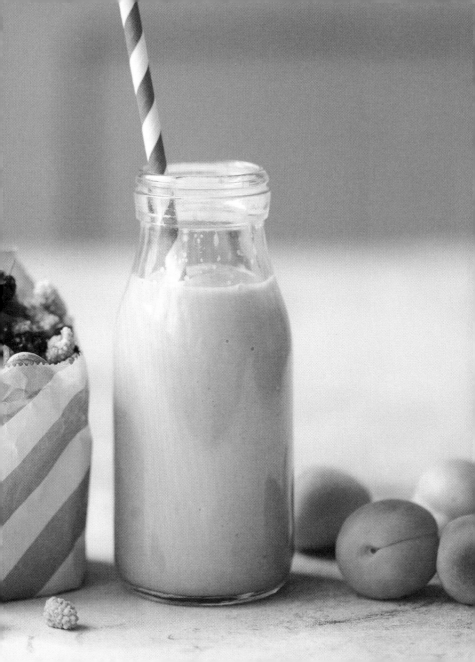

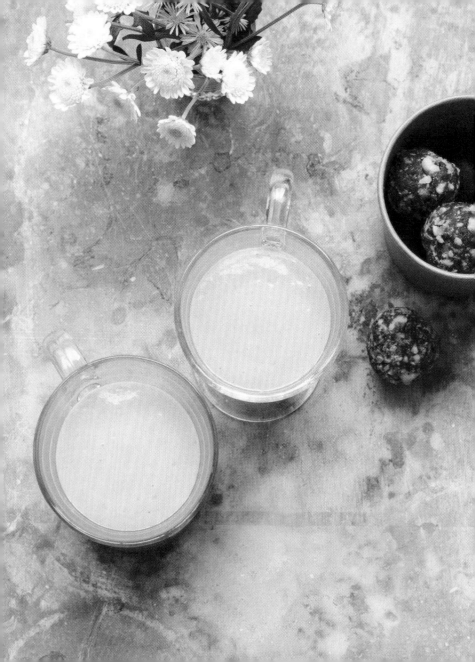

BANANA &
MATCHA SMOOTHIE

This matcha smoothie is a lovely breakfast option, made with banana, spinach and almond milk, it's a really great way to start your day. I normally leave the dates out, as I quite like my morning smoothies not to be too sweet and the banana usually gives the right level of sweetness for me, but feel free to add them in, if you need them to enjoy it – remember, it's so much better to adjust the recipe if it means you'll enjoy every sip. Without the dates it's not that sweet, so if you're not ready for something more green, try with the dates first.

SERVES 1

¼ ripe avocado (40g)

1 ripe banana, peeled and frozen (100g)

½ teaspoon matcha green tea powder

handful of fresh or frozen spinach (about 30g, but adjust depending on how green you like it!)

¾ glass of chilled almond milk, or any other plant-based milk (300ml)

1–2 medjool dates, pitted and chopped (optional)

Pit and peel the avocado, then put it into a blender.

Add all the remaining ingredients and blend until smooth and creamy.

TIP Cut medjool dates into quarters before blending, so they mix properly, otherwise you'll be left with little clumps at the bottom of your cup! If you don't want to use medjool dates (as they are more expensive), then you can use regular dates, just make sure they're soft enough to blend. If they're not, soak them in warm water to soften before using.

MANGO, LIME & KALE

This smoothie tastes so fresh and green, but still really creamy, with sweet fruity hints in each sip. I love using the cashews and almond milk to create a lovely thick texture and the ginger and lime to add a little spicy, zesty element, which – alongside the mango – helps to balance out the flavour of the kale.

SERVES 1

small chunk of fresh ginger (18g)
½ ripe mango (170g)
handful of kale (30g, or adjust depending on how green you want it!)
juice of ½ lime
½ glass of chilled almond milk (200ml)
handful of cashews (35g)

Peel the ginger. Peel and pit the mango, and tear off and discard any coarse ribs from the kale leaves.

Put everything into a blender and blend until smooth and creamy. This may take a little longer than some of the other smoothies, as cashew nuts can take longer to break up, depending on the strength of your blender.

TIP Using frozen fruit is the best way to make your smoothie cold without having to water it down using lots of ice. This way the flavour and texture are so much better, and you can always add a few cubes of ice to the glass at the end if you want it to be really chilled and refreshing.

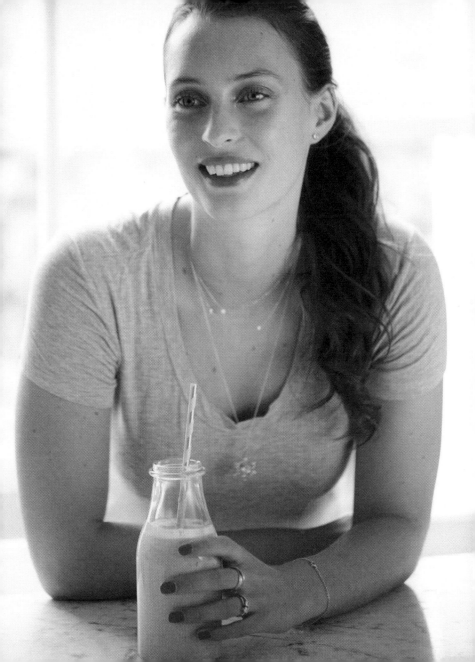

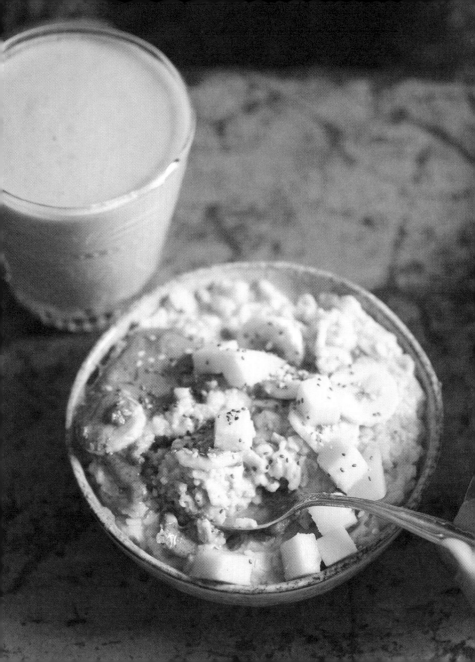

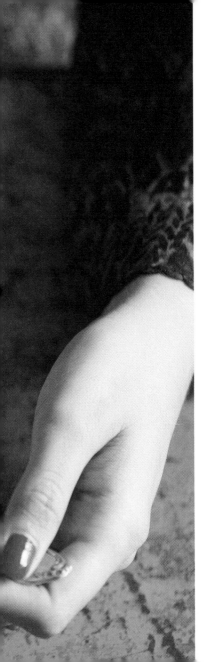

TURMERIC & GINGER

A great pick-me-up, this smoothie is my go-to when I'm feeling a bit run-down. The ginger and turmeric really boost me, while the orange, mango, sesame and banana give it such a lovely flavour. If you want to sweeten it you can add a squeeze of honey or a date, but I think it tastes fantastic just like this. If you can't find fresh turmeric, use ground, though fresh tastes much better!

NUT FREE

SERVES 1

1 orange (150g)
½ mango (170g)
½ ripe banana, peeled and frozen
  (about 50g)
6g fresh turmeric, peeled, or
  ½ teaspoon ground turmeric
½ glass of chilled plant-based milk,
  I like coconut milk (200ml)
1.5cm piece of ginger, peeled
1 teaspoon sesame seeds

Juice the orange. Peel and pit the mango. Put both into a blender.

Add all the other ingredients and blend until completely smooth.

CARROT CAKE SMOOTHIE

This may sound a bit bizarre, but trust me, it's so delicious! It's one of the most dessert-like recipes in the book, as it's so sweet and creamy with lots of spices. I love it for breakfast, but it's also fun in little glasses as snacks for friends when they come over.

SERVES 1

1 ripe banana, peeled and frozen
  (about 100g)
70g pineapple chunks, frozen
1 small carrot, peeled and chopped (50g)
½ glass of chilled almond milk (200ml)
1 medjool date, pitted and chopped
1 teaspoon ground cinnamon
pinch of ground ginger
pinch of ground nutmeg
1 teaspoon vanilla powder
1 teaspoon cashew butter
squeeze of honey (optional)

Simply place everything in a blender and blend until smooth.

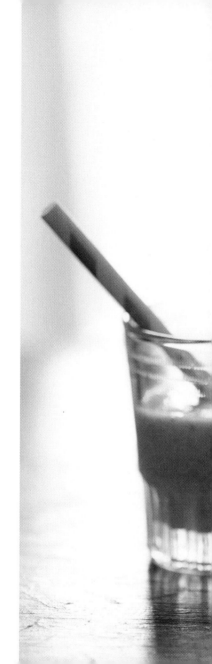

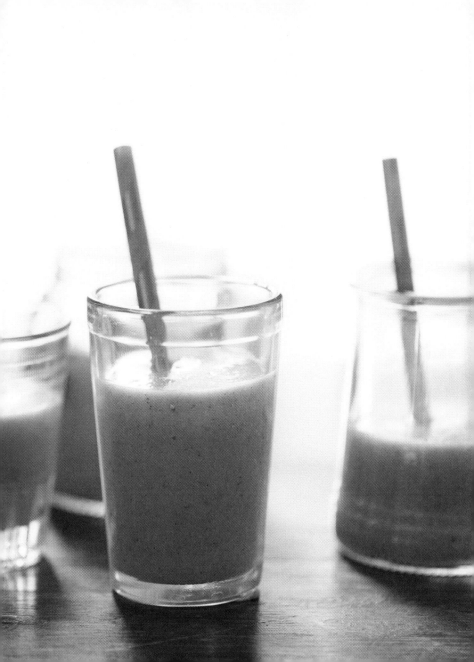

ICED MINT & MATCHA LATTE

This is the best cooling drink on a hot day, or an energising accompaniment to any meal. I'll often make one of these with lunch to sip on as I munch through my meal. The mint adds a lovely freshness and I find it's perfect without the honey but if you like it a little sweeter, feel free to blend it in.

SERVES 1

½ teaspoon matcha green tea powder
about 5 fresh mint leaves
½–1 teaspoon honey (optional)
¾ glass of chilled almond milk, or any
   other plant-based milk (300ml)
good handful of ice cubes

Put the matcha, mint, honey (if using) and almond milk into a blender with a few ice cubes, then whizz until smooth and creamy.

Pour the drink over ice cubes to serve.

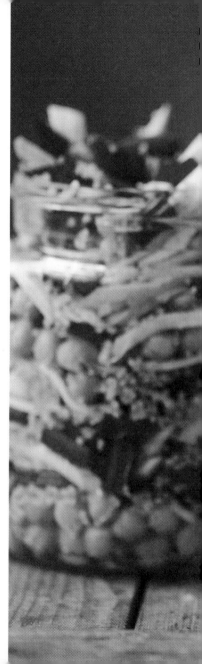

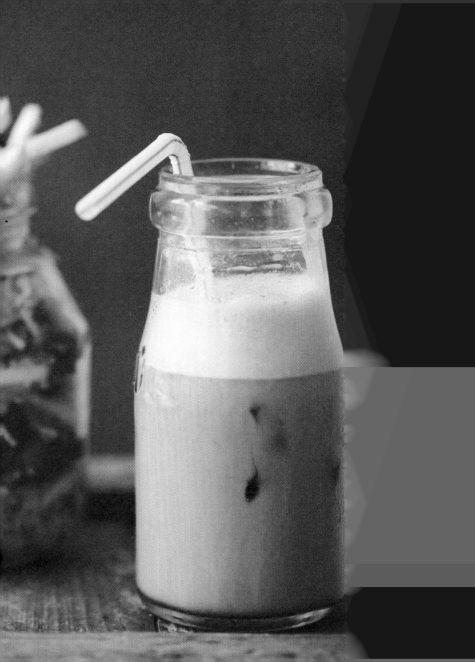

MINTY COCONUT SHAKE

This is a regular treat when I want to sate my sweet tooth. I often make this in the afternoons, or after a meal, when I want quite a light drink, so I leave the banana out. But if you want a thick, creamy smoothie then definitely add it in, or use half an avocado instead. I'm sure this will become a favourite of yours, too!

SERVES 1

¾ glass of chilled coconut water, preferably raw and unpasteurised (300ml)
1 teaspoon coconut oil
3 medjool dates, pitted and chopped
squeeze of lime juice
small handful of fresh mint (10g)
1 heaped teaspoon cashew butter
1 ripe banana, peeled and frozen (100g), or ½ avocado, peeled and pitted (80g), both optional

Place everything in a blender and blend until smooth.

CREAMY CARAMEL & VANILLA

A dessert-style smoothie. Dates and maca give a caramel-like flavour, while vanilla adds lovely sweetness. I add avocado to up the greens and give a smooth texture, and coconut water to stop it from being too rich, but for something extra-indulgent, use creamy hazelnut milk instead.

NUT FREE
SERVES 1

½ ripe avocado (80g)
½ glass of chilled coconut water, preferably raw and unpasteurised (200ml)
2 medjool dates, pitted and chopped
1 teaspoon cacao powder
1 teaspoon maca powder
1 teaspoon vanilla powder
squeeze of honey (optional)

Pit and peel the avocado, then put it into a blender with all the remaining ingredients except the honey and blend until smooth and creamy. I'd recommend tasting it before deciding if it needs honey, as I'm sure lots of you will think it's great as it is.

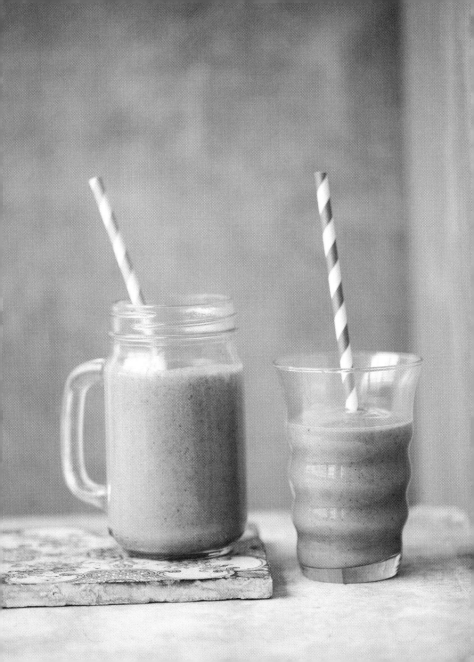

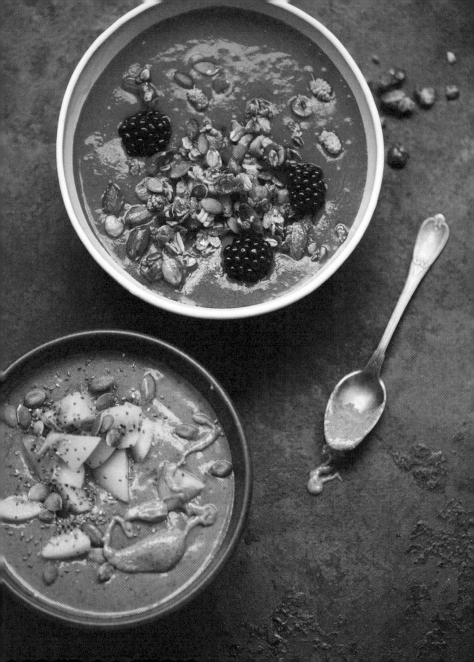

AÇAI BOWLS TWO WAYS

Açai bowls are a favourite weekend breakfast of mine, as they're sweet and creamy and can be loaded up with so many toppings. I love piling mine high with everything I have in my cupboard, from home-made granola to chunks of energy bites, fresh fruit, nuts, seeds and anything else I have floating around! The beet version may sound weirder than the coconut, but trust me, it's worth being open-minded about it as it tastes so good! For this drink, it's even more important than usual that the bananas are super-ripe, as it makes a tremendous difference to the taste.

TIP You can find frozen açai pulp and frozen coconut meat online or in health food shops. For the coconut, you should look for young coconut meat. If you can't find it, don't worry, just scoop the flesh out of a coconut shell after you drink the water, seal it in a freezer bag and freeze it yourself.

NUT FREE (CREAMY COCONUT)

EACH MAKES 1 BOWL

FOR A CREAMY COCONUT AÇAI
110g frozen açai pulp (see Tip, left)
60g frozen coconut meat (see Tip, left)
¼ glass of chilled coconut milk (100ml)
2 teaspoons chia seeds
25g blueberries

FOR A SWEET BEET AÇAI
110g frozen açai pulp (see Tip, left)
1 small raw beetroot, peeled and roughly chopped (110g)
1 very ripe banana, peeled and frozen (100g)
1 teaspoon almond butter
¼ glass of chilled almond milk (100ml)
juice of 1 lime

For both bowls, simply place all the ingredients in a blender and blend until thick and creamy, like soft-serve ice cream.

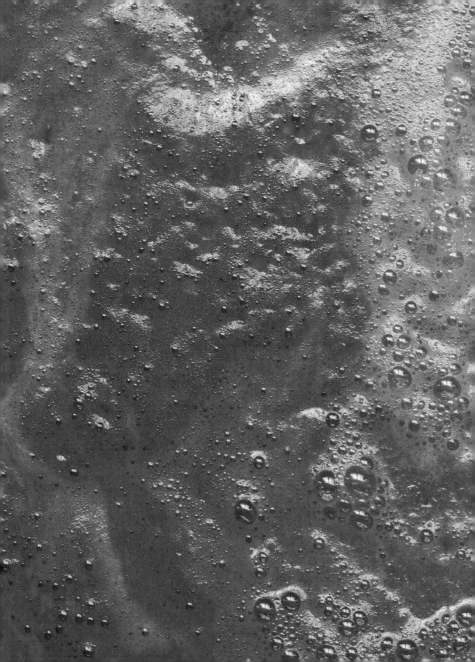

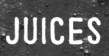

JUICES

JUICES INTRO

This chapter will take you through all my favourite juices. First, I want to talk a bit about juicing, and share some of my tips and tricks.

Juices are an amazing way to sneak a little goodness into your day, plus they're so delicious. I normally go for green-based juices, as I find it's the quickest way to ramp up my intake of greens, but there are lots of other options for those of you who aren't ready to start drinking celery and fennel just yet! (I certainly wasn't ready for those on day one, either...)

This may sound obvious, but if you're new to juicing, it's important to quickly note that juices are made using a juicer, rather than a blender. This is a machine designed just for juicing and the process removes most of the fibrous part of the fruit and veg, to create a thin liquid.

Unlike blenders, you can't put everything into a juicer, as some produce won't give you a great yield, so it can feel like a waste of good food. You want to use ingredients that fill your glass up without you having to buy kilos and kilos of them! Hard fruit and veg like apples, pears, carrots, beets and fennel work really well, as do those with a high water content like cucumber, celery, watermelon and citrus fruit. You can also add spices and herbs, like ginger, mint, parsley and coriander. (I leave things like bananas, mangos and avocados for my blender.)

As a result, I sometimes find myself making half-smoothies and half-juices, and you'll discover some of those in this chapter. I'll juice some cucumber, for instance, then blend it with banana, nut butter and so on to get the best of both worlds.

Blending in your leafy greens works well, too, as you don't always get a particularly high juice yield from things like spinach and kale. You can try doing this with any juice; if you're new to the process and starting with fruitier juices, then try throwing the juices in the blender with some spinach. It won't affect the taste much, but it will increase your veggie intake. It's worth pointing out that your beautifully vibrant, pink juice may go swamp-coloured when doing this, so it won't look as appealing but – I promise – it affects the look of a drink much more than the taste!

TYPES OF JUICERS

There are lots of different types of juicers: the main ones are masticating, centrifugal and cold-press. As picking one can be a bit confusing, I wanted to quickly share what these words mean.

Masticating juicers juice the produce slowly and are designed to let it pass through without heating it. They turn and push the ingredients through, slowly crushing them, rather than grinding them, which is what a centrifugal juicer does.

The centrifugal method is used in most juicers; it's fast and efficient, and these machines often have much bigger feed tubes so you can drop in lots of produce at once, often whole, which means it's a speedier process for you. A centrifugal juicer is what I use at home.

Cold-press juicers aren't generally used at home, as they're unbelievably expensive and are mostly used in commercial juice bars. We have one at the Mae Deli.

My biggest piece of advice would be to buy a juicer that's easy to clean. They tend to have lots of parts, so I would pick one where everything can go into your dishwasher!

TIP Try to store all your juice ingredients in the fridge so that they're cold when they are put through the juicer. This will keep the juice chilled, without you having to water it down with lots of ice.

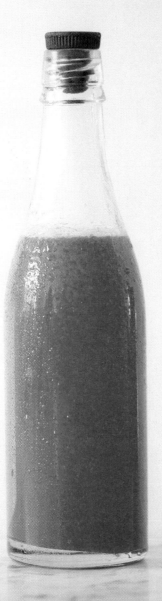

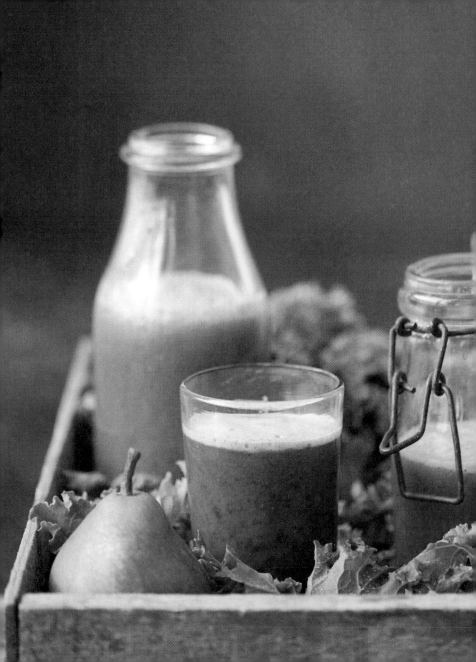

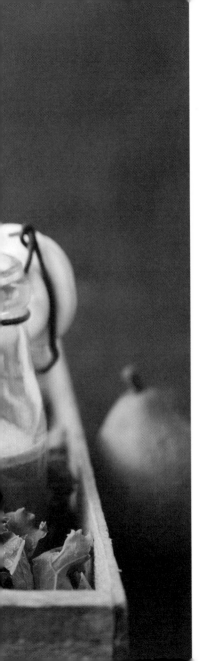

EASY GREEN

This easy green blend is a great way to start your juice journey. The mix of pear and apple balances out the cucumber and kale perfectly, making each sip nicely sweet but still filled with greens. This way you can get used to the idea of drinking veg without it feeling too weird! One of the first juices I made... and I still love it.

NUT FREE

SERVES 1

¾ cucumber (255g)
handful of kale (30g)
1 pear (180g)
1 apple (150g)

Work everything through a juicer. I find I get most from the kale when I juice it with the other ingredients, rather than doing it at the end.

TIP Whisk superfood powders, like maca, into your juice at the end to add more flavour.

SWEET GREEN

This is one of my absolute favourite recipes. I adore pineapple, so any recipe with it in always makes me so happy. Adding the cooling cucumber tastes amazing, while the ginger gives it a great kick and the lime adds a zesty element. Another great 'beginner's' green juice, you can always adjust the ratio of pineapple to cucumber to make it sweeter or more green, depending on your taste buds.

NUT FREE

SERVES 1

⅓ pineapple (300g)
thumb-sized piece of ginger (30g)
½ lime (20g)
1 cucumber (340g)

Peel and roughly chop the pineapple. Peel the ginger. Peel the lime, making sure to remove all the white pith.

Work everything through a juicer. I find I get more from the ginger when I juice it with the cucumber or pineapple, rather than doing it at the end.

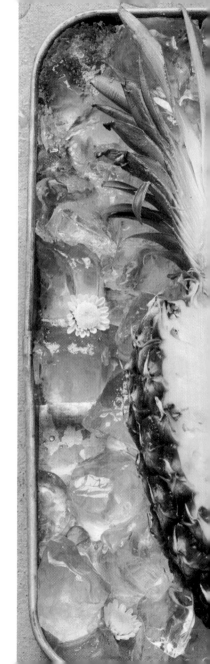

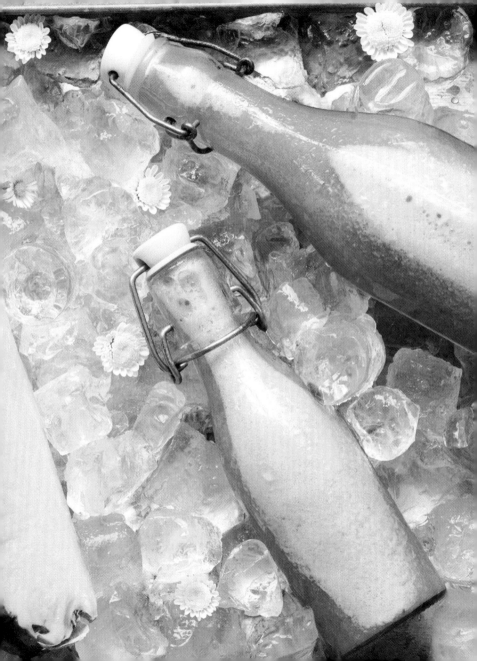

HERBY GREEN

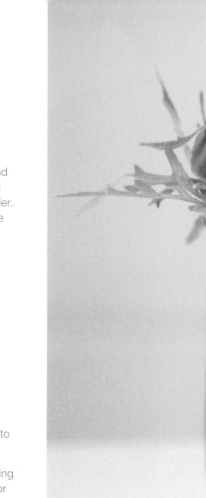

This herby green blend is a lovely way to start a morning. I head for this juice when I've eaten lots of sweet things and am craving some greens. It may sound a bit weird to drink parsley and coriander, but I promise it doesn't taste as strange as it sounds! As with the other all-veg mixes, feel free to add some apple to sweeten this.

NUT FREE

SERVES 1

1 lemon (60g)
1 cucumber (340g)
small handful of fresh parsley (15g)
small handful of fresh coriander (15g)
3 celery sticks (135g)

Carefully peel the lemon, making sure to remove all the white pith.

Work everything through a juicer, passing the herbs through with the cucumber or celery, rather than doing them at the end, for the best result.

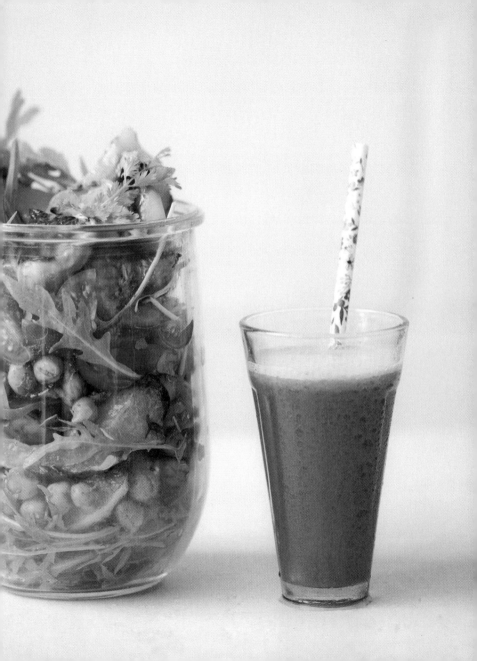

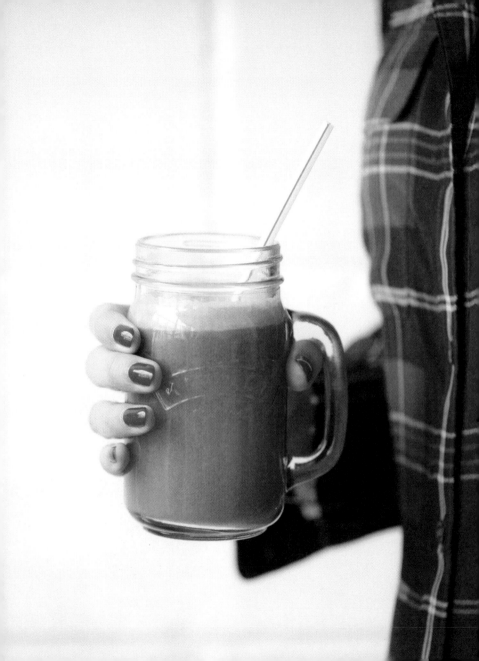

FENNEL & MINT

Adding the fennel, mint and lime to this all-veg mix is such a nice way to lighten the flavour and add a little sweetness; you'll still feel very virtuous drinking your broccoli, though! This is the freshest tasting of the all-green juice recipes in this book, so I normally make this one in the afternoons and serve it with lots of ice.

NUT FREE

SERVES 1

½ lime (20g)
½ fennel bulb (140g)
small handful of fresh mint (15g)
large handful of spinach (40g)
1¼ cucumbers (425g)
½ head of broccoli (200g)

Carefully peel the lime, making sure to remove all the white pith.

Work everything through a juicer. I find I get the most juice from the mint and spinach when I juice them with the cucumber or celery, rather than doing them at the end.

DEEP GREEN

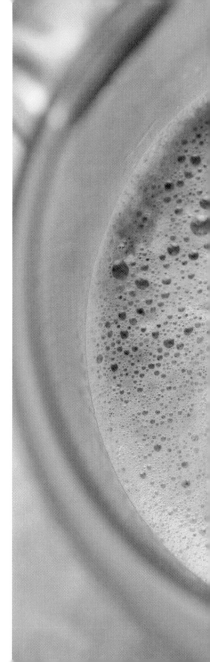

This is one of my go-to green juices. As with Herby Green and Fennel & Mint (see pages 52 and 55) it's mostly veg, but the lemon gives it a lovely flavour and the cucumber makes it really refreshing. Feel free to take out some of the cucumber and add an apple, though, if you want to sweeten it – that's how I first started making this combination.

NUT FREE

SERVES 1

½ lemon (30g)
large handful of spinach (40g)
handful of kale (30g)
1¼ cucumbers (425g)
1 celery stick (45g)

Carefully peel the lemon, making sure to remove all the white pith.

Work everything through a juicer, juicing the leafy greens at the same time as the cucumbers and celery for the best result.

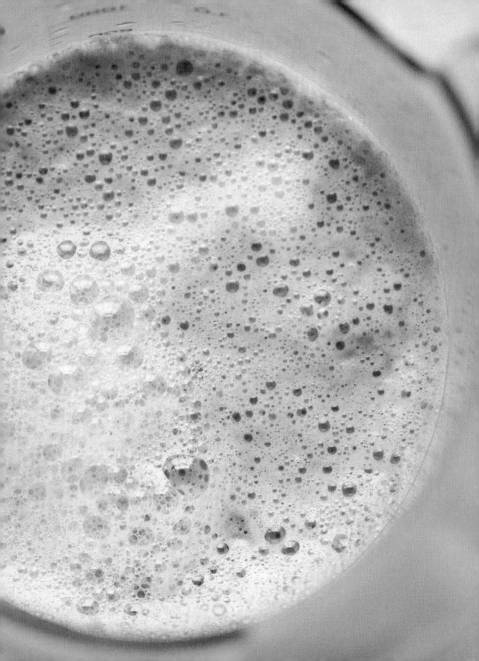

SPICY TOMATO

Probably the most savoury juice in the book. It's more of a lunch/dinner/snack accompaniment than a breakfast for most people, but it's one of the most delicious mixes here and I couldn't recommend it more! The blend of juicy tomato, celery and cucumber with tamari, apple cider vinegar and cayenne is such a winner.

NUT FREE

SERVES 1

4 tomatoes (480g)
1 lemon (60g)
⅓ large cucumber (150g)
2 celery sticks (90g)
1 teaspoon tamari
1 teaspoon apple cider vinegar
sprinkle of cayenne pepper
salt and pepper

Halve the tomatoes and scoop out the seeds. Carefully peel the lemon, making sure to remove all the white pith.

Work the tomatoes and lemon through a juicer with the cucumber and celery. Then stir in the tamari, vinegar and cayenne and season with salt and pepper.

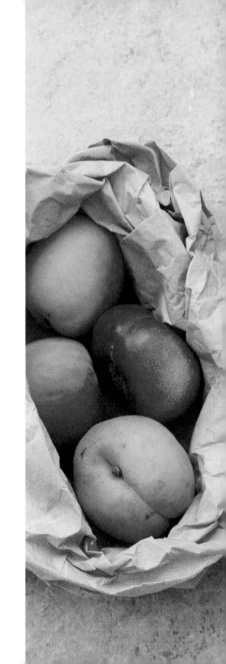

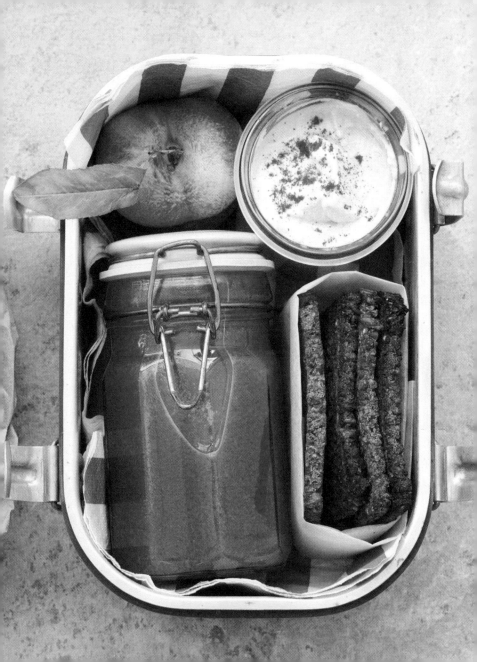

ORANGE, SWEET POTATO & CARROT

This blend, with carrot, orange, ginger, lemon and lemon grass, is such a lovely take on a classic carrot and ginger juice. It adds so many more flavours to create a really rich blend that has the perfect amount of sweetness.

NUT FREE

SERVES 1

1 sweet potato (270g)
small thumb-sized piece of ginger (22g)
thumb-sized piece of fresh turmeric (22g)
1 orange (150g)
½ lemon (30g)
1 stalk of lemon grass (12g)
5 carrots (400g)

Peel the sweet potato, ginger and turmeric. Carefully peel both the orange and lemon, making sure to remove all the white pith.

Work everything through a juicer. I'd recommend putting the ginger, turmeric and lemon grass through with the bigger items towards the start, to get the most from them.

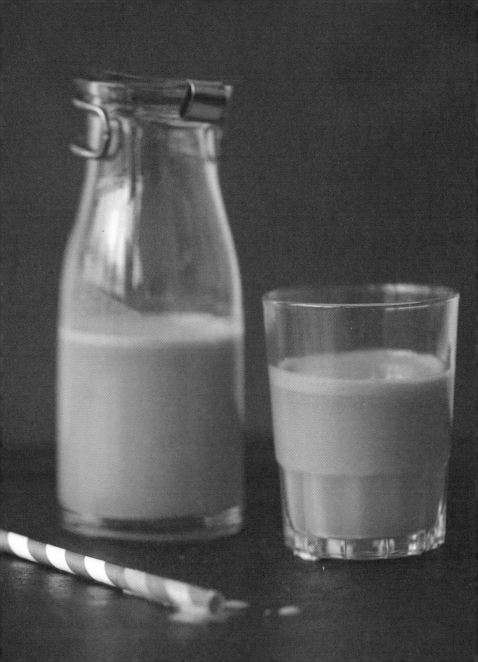

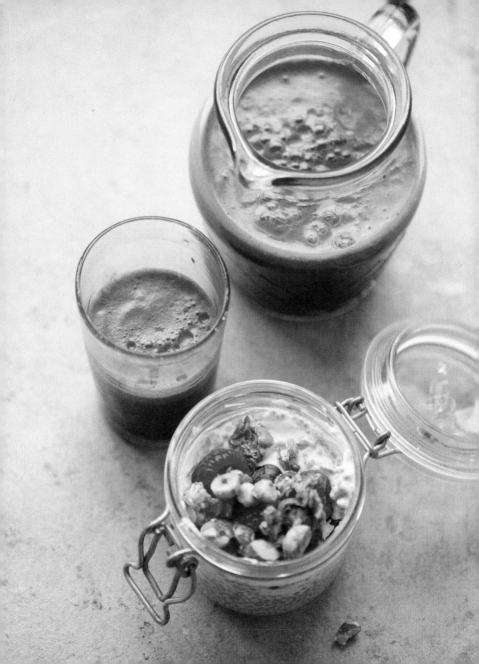

BEET, CARROT & GINGER

Beet juice is one of my favourite things, I just love the vibrant pink colour. The carrot, apple and lime here balance the earthy nature of the beets with their sweetness, while the cucumber and parsley make the drink taste really fresh.

NUT FREE

SERVES 1

2 small beetroots (220g)
big thumb-sized piece of ginger (35g)
¼ lime (10g)
a few sprigs of fresh parsley (5g)
4 carrots (340g)
½ cucumber (170g)
1 small apple (110g)

Peel the beetroots and ginger and carefully peel the lime, making sure to remove all the white pith.

Work everything through a juicer, adding the parsley at the same time as some of the veg for the best result.

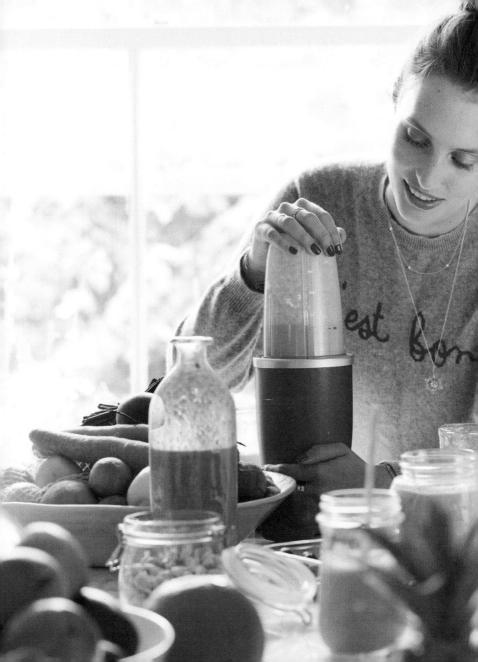

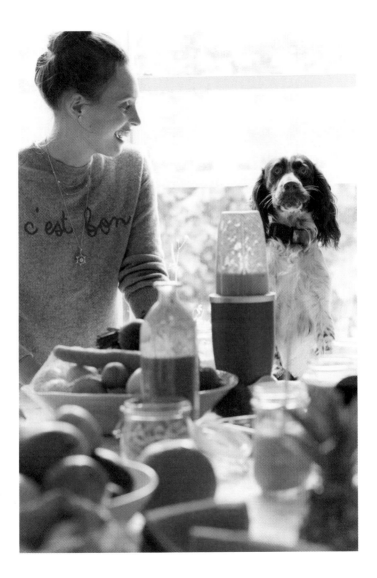

MELON & MINT

This is the perfect summer drink; it's sweet and cooling with lovely hints of mint among the melon, watermelon, cucumber and red grapes. If you're looking to get your friends and family interested in juicing, these blends of fruit with herbs and cucumber can be a good place to start, as they're absolutely delicious and not green and scary at all!

NUT FREE

SERVES 1

¼ honeydew melon (245g)
small chunk of watermelon (200g)
small handful of fresh mint (10g)
¼ cucumber (85g)
small bunch of red grapes (135g),
   stalks discarded

Remove the rind from both melons, de-seed and roughly chop.

Work everything through a juicer, adding the mint at the same time as the other ingredients to get the most from it.

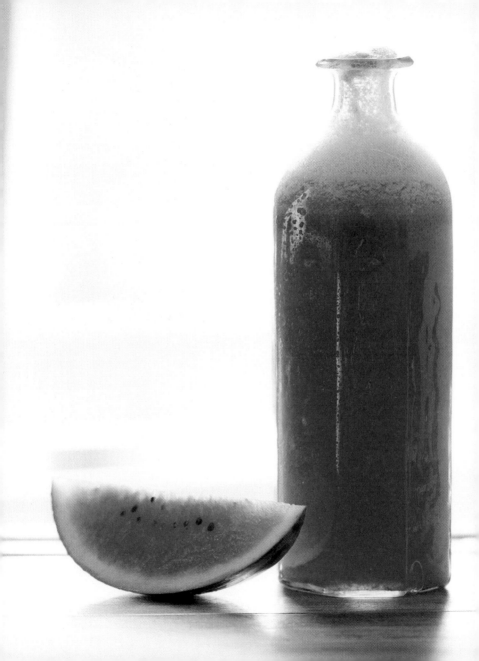

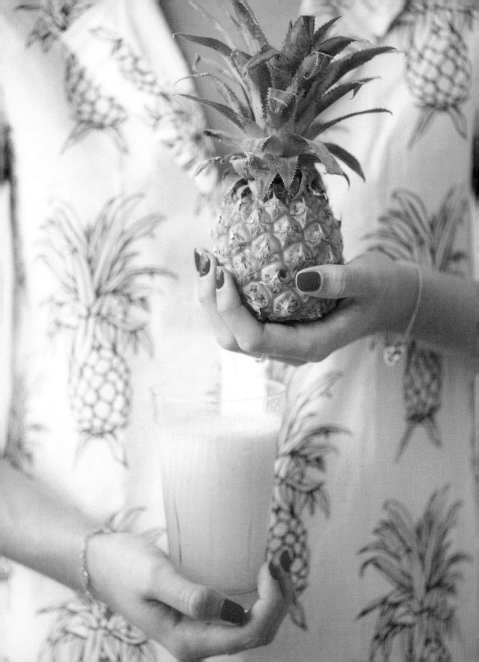

SPICED PINEAPPLE & PASSION FRUIT

This juice – with its hits of lime, ginger and mint – is a real winner. It's one of my favourite afternoon snacks, especially in the summer. It tastes perfect on a warm day, served with lots of ice and shared with friends.

NUT FREE

SERVES 1

⅔ pineapple (570g)
big thumb-sized piece of ginger (40g)
½ lime (20g)
3 passion fruits (weight of flesh
    scooped out of skin, 80g)
small handful of fresh mint (10g)

Peel and roughly chop the pineapple. Peel the ginger. Carefully peel the lime, making sure to remove all the white pith. Scoop the flesh out of the passion fruits.

Work everything through a juicer, adding the mint and ginger at the same time as the other ingredients, as that way it will be easiest to get the most flavour from them.

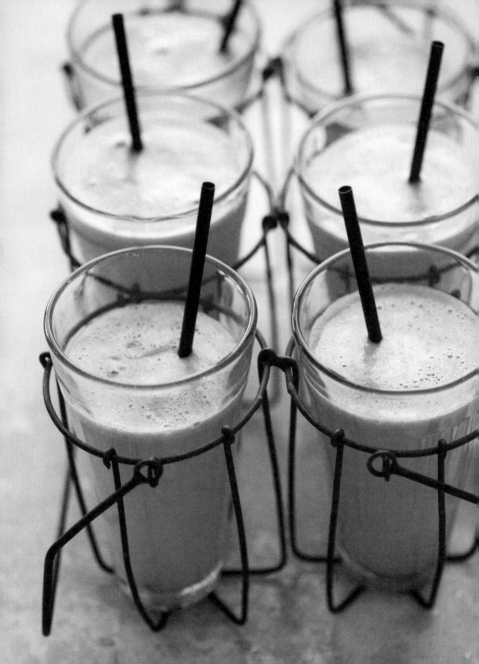

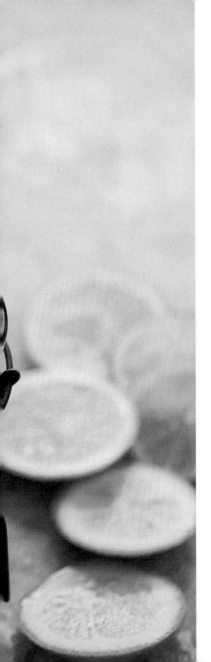

TRIPLE CITRUS

This citrus juice is perfect for those of you who love orange juice and are looking for a more exciting way to make it. Adding the grapefruit, lime and lemon grass means the classic juice has a whole new range of flavours that I'm sure you'll all love!

NUT FREE

SERVES 1

1½ oranges (225g)
1 grapefruit (350g)
1 lime (40g)
1 stalk of lemon grass (12g)

Carefully peel the oranges, grapefruit and lime, making sure to remove all the white pith from each.

Work everything through a juicer, making sure the lemon grass is juiced towards the beginning of the process.

TIP I normally make my juice and drink it straight away, but it can be stored in an airtight container for up to two days. It will separate during this time though, so give it a good shake before drinking.

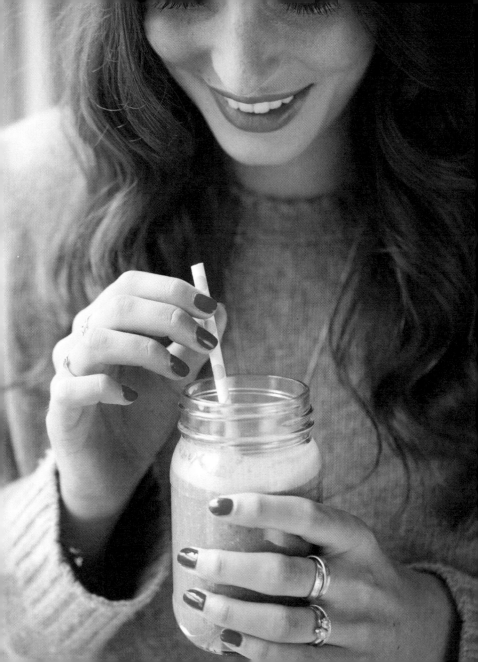

SWEET & CREAMY CUCUMBER & APPLE

Using juice as the base for a smoothie is fantastic, as you get the best of both worlds. This is one of my favourite recipes using the two methods; it's a great way to start juicing too, as it feels more accessible. The banana and dates in this recipe make it lovely and sweet, while the almond butter makes it nice and creamy.

SERVES 1

⅔ cucumber (230g)
1½ large apples (180g)
handful of spinach (30g)
1 ripe banana, peeled and frozen
  (100g)
1 tablespoon almond butter
2 medjool dates, pitted and chopped

Juice the cucumber and apples to make your base.

Pour the juice into a blender with all the remaining ingredients and blend until smooth and creamy.

TIP When I make juice for the juice–smoothie blends, I often make three servings at once, then keep them in an airtight container in the fridge. That way I save time the next few mornings.

MANGO, GINGER
& CUCUMBER

This blend is so delicious. Using cucumber in the base juice adds a lovely refreshing element to each sip, while the avocado and mango make it really creamy. I love the flavours of the ginger, lime and honey with this too, perfect for an energising breakfast or afternoon pick-me-up.

NUT FREE

SERVES 1

½ lime (20g)
1 cucumber (340g)
½ avocado (80g)
a few chunks of mango (50g)
slice of peeled ginger (8g)
1 teaspoon honey

Carefully peel the lime, making sure to remove all the white pith. Juice the cucumber and lime, then pour the juice into a blender.

Pit and peel the avocado and the mango. Add everything to the blender and blend until smooth.

TIP Juice pulp from your juicer can be hard to re-use, as most of the flavour has been taken out already. I find it's best baked into crackers with lots of seasoning, or used as compost for your garden.

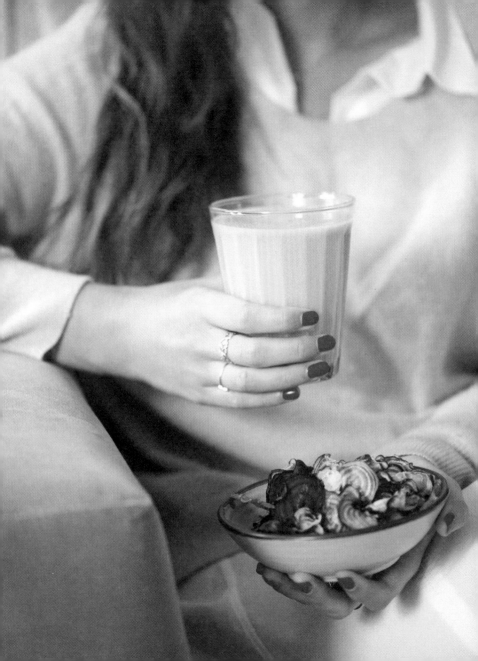

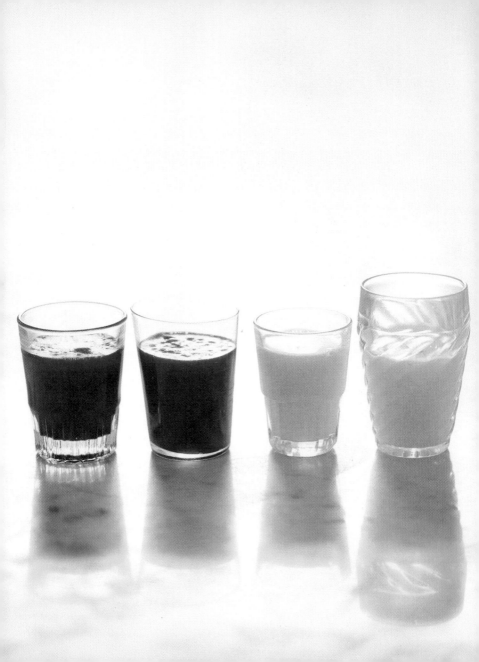

SHOTS

These little juice shots are great ways to start the day. They always wake me up and help me begin the morning in the best way, especially when I'm feeling a bit run down. You can make a couple at a time and store them in airtight containers in the fridge to enjoy over two days. I go for the Pick-me-up when I'm feeling a cold coming on, and The Reviver when I'm really exhausted.

THE REVIVER
NUT FREE
SERVES 3

2 small beetroots (220g)
1 lemon (60g)
small handful of fresh mint (10g)

Peel the beets. Carefully peel the lemon, making sure to remove all the white pith.

Work everything through a juicer, adding the mint at the same time as the other ingredients.

PICK-ME-UP
NUT FREE
SERVES 3

2 lemons (120g)
big knob of ginger (75g)
1 tablespoon apple cider vinegar
1 teaspoon honey
sprinkle of cayenne pepper

Carefully peel the lemons, making sure to remove all the white pith. Peel the ginger.

Work the lemons and ginger through a juicer at the same time.

Stir in all the remaining ingredients.

INDEX

First published in Great Britain in 2016 by Yellow Kite
An imprint of Hodder & Stoughton
An Hachette UK company
1

A CIP catalogue record for this title is available
from the British Library

Hardback ISBN 978 1 47364 7282
eBook ISBN 978 1 47364 7299

Publisher: Liz Gough
Design and Art Direction: Miranda Harvey
Photography: Clare Winfield
Photo Shoot Co-ordinator: Ruth Ferrier
Food stylist: Eleanor Mulligan
Props stylist: Polly Webb-Wilson
Make-up Artist: Laurey Simmons

Printed and bound in Italy by Lego SpA

Hodder & Stoughton policy is to use papers that
are natural, renewable and recyclable products and
made from wood grown in sustainable forests. The
logging and manufacturing processes are expected
to conform to the environmental regulations of the
country of origin.

Yellow Kite
Hodder & Stoughton Ltd
Carmelite House
50 Victoria Embankment
London EC4Y 0DZ

www.yellowkitebooks.co.uk
www.hodder.co.uk

The advice herein is not intended
to replace the services of trained
health professionals, or to be a
substitute for medical advice.
You are advised to consult with
your health care professional with
regard to matters relating to your
health, and in particular regarding
matters that may require
diagnosis or medical attention.

For more amazing recipes and
inspiration from Deliciously Ella,
look out for her original bestsellers
Deliciously Ella and *Deliciously Ella
Every Day*, available now from all
good book shops and online, and
the exciting upcoming *Deliciously
Ella With Friends*, out January 2017.

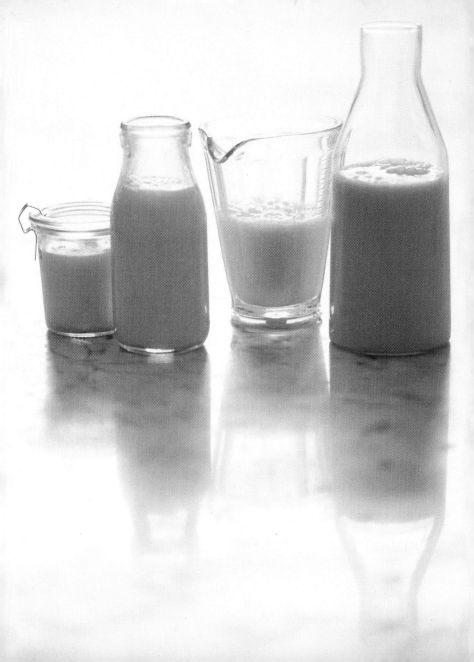